BEING ME IS Special

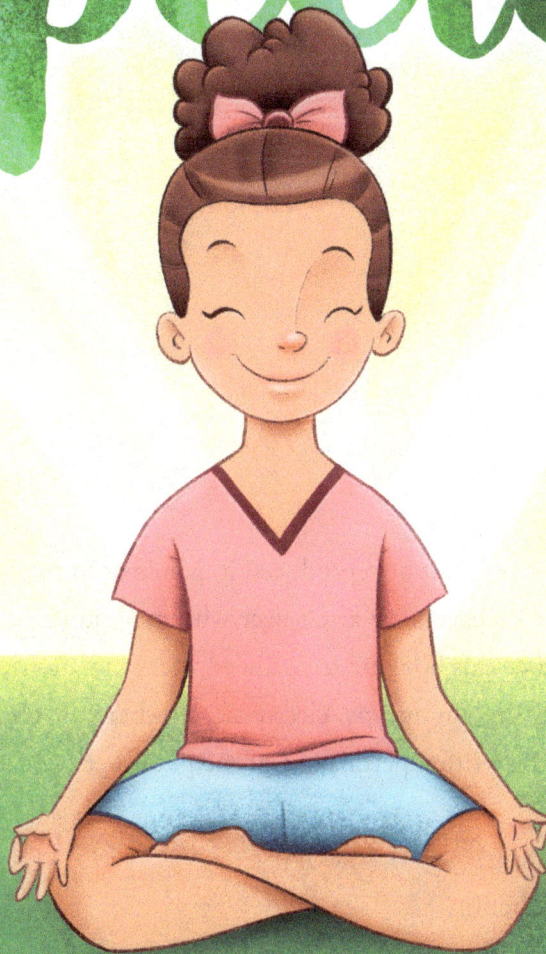

A celebration of movement and mindfulness through yoga

TOMMIE BURCH | ILLUSTRATED BY Nate Myers

ISBN: 979-8-218-52678-8 (Print)
ISBN: 979-8-218-52679-5 (Ebook)

Design and Illustrations: Nate Myers, https://nwmyers.com

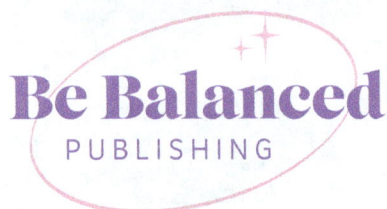

Be Balanced
PUBLISHING

To my daughter,
May you always love yourself fiercely.
You are smart, you are kind, you are strong, and
you can do anything you want in this world.

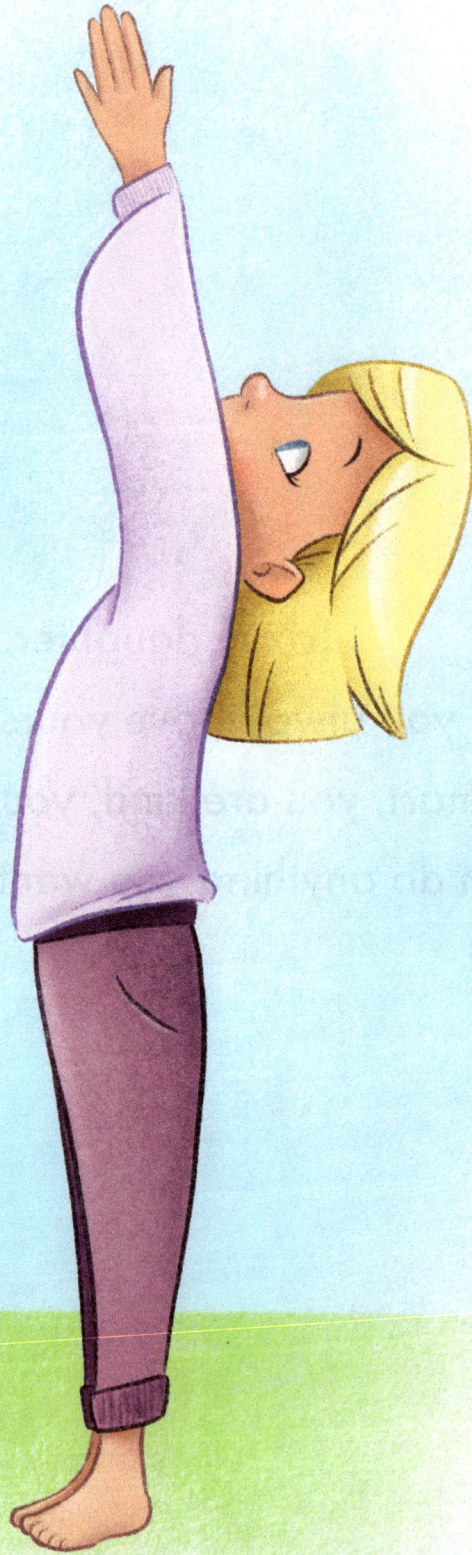

BEING ME IS SPECIAL,

from my toes up to my crown.

BEING ME IS SPECIAL

when I'm up and when I'm down.

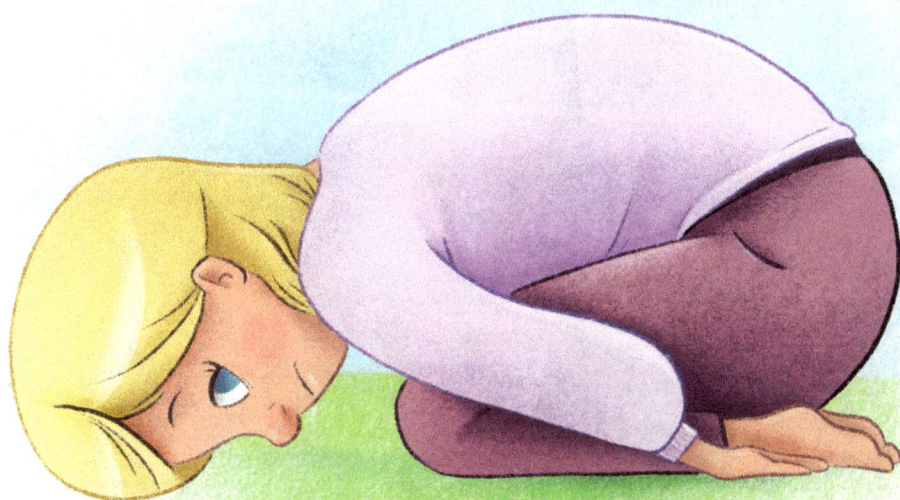

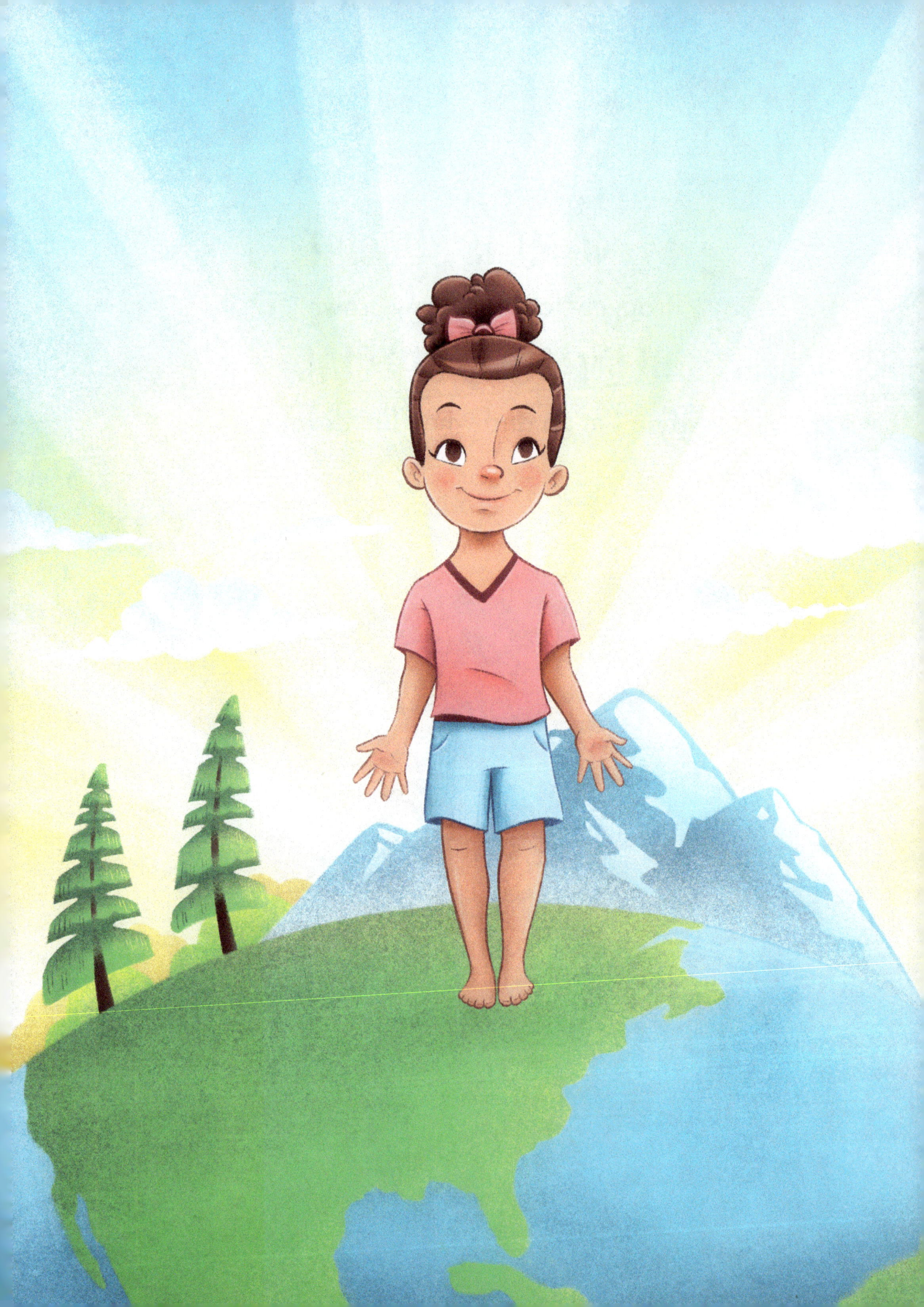

I LOVE MY STEADY FEET ...

they feel the earth below.

I say **THANK YOU** to my feet

when I stand in Mountain pose.

I LOVE MY BIG, STRONG LEGS . . .

they help me run and play.

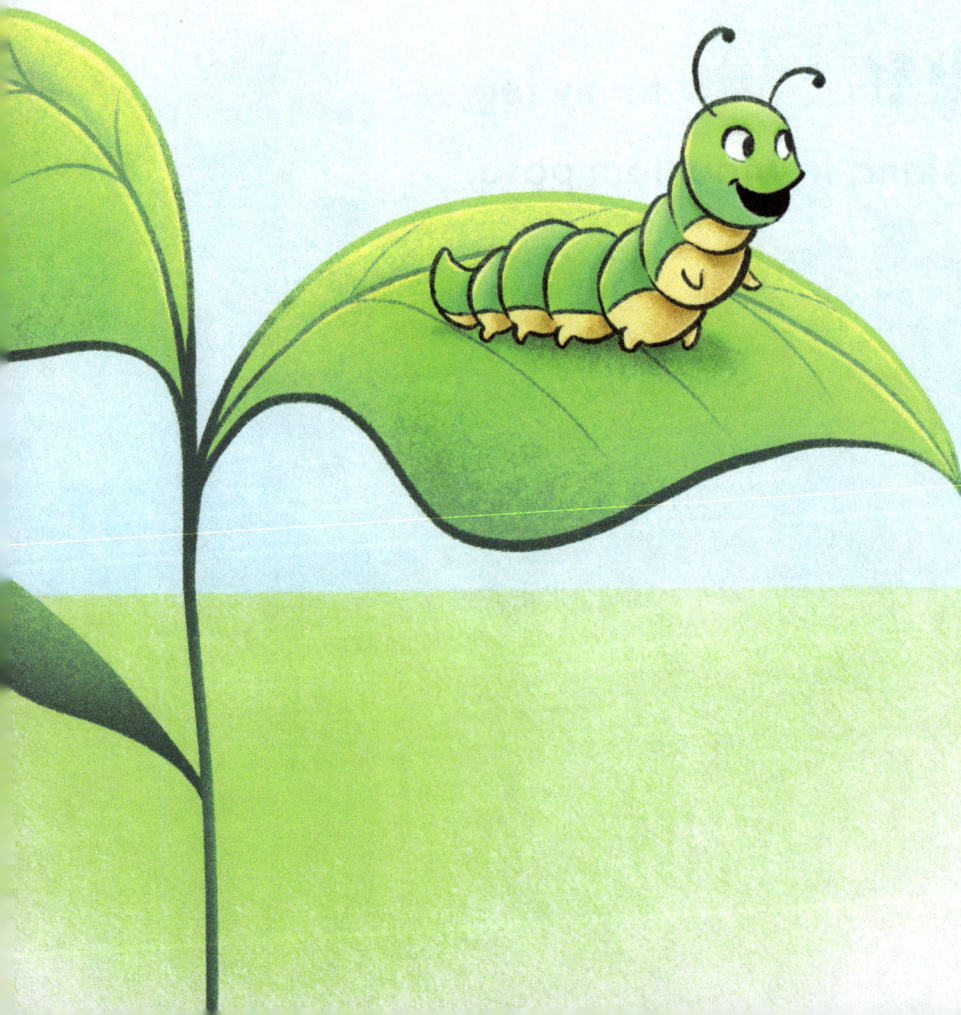

I stretch my legs in Staff pose.
I THANK THEM EVERY DAY.

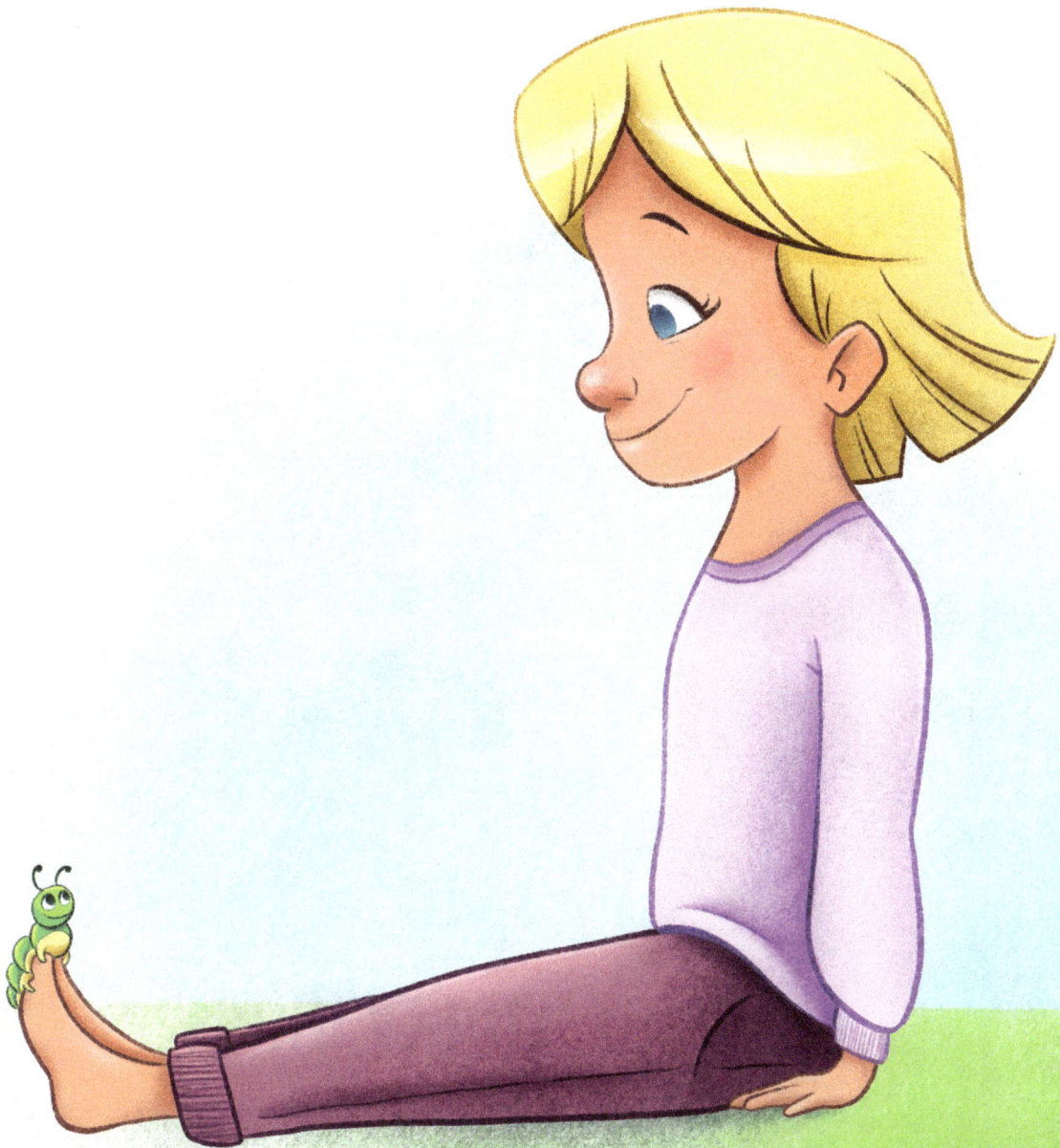

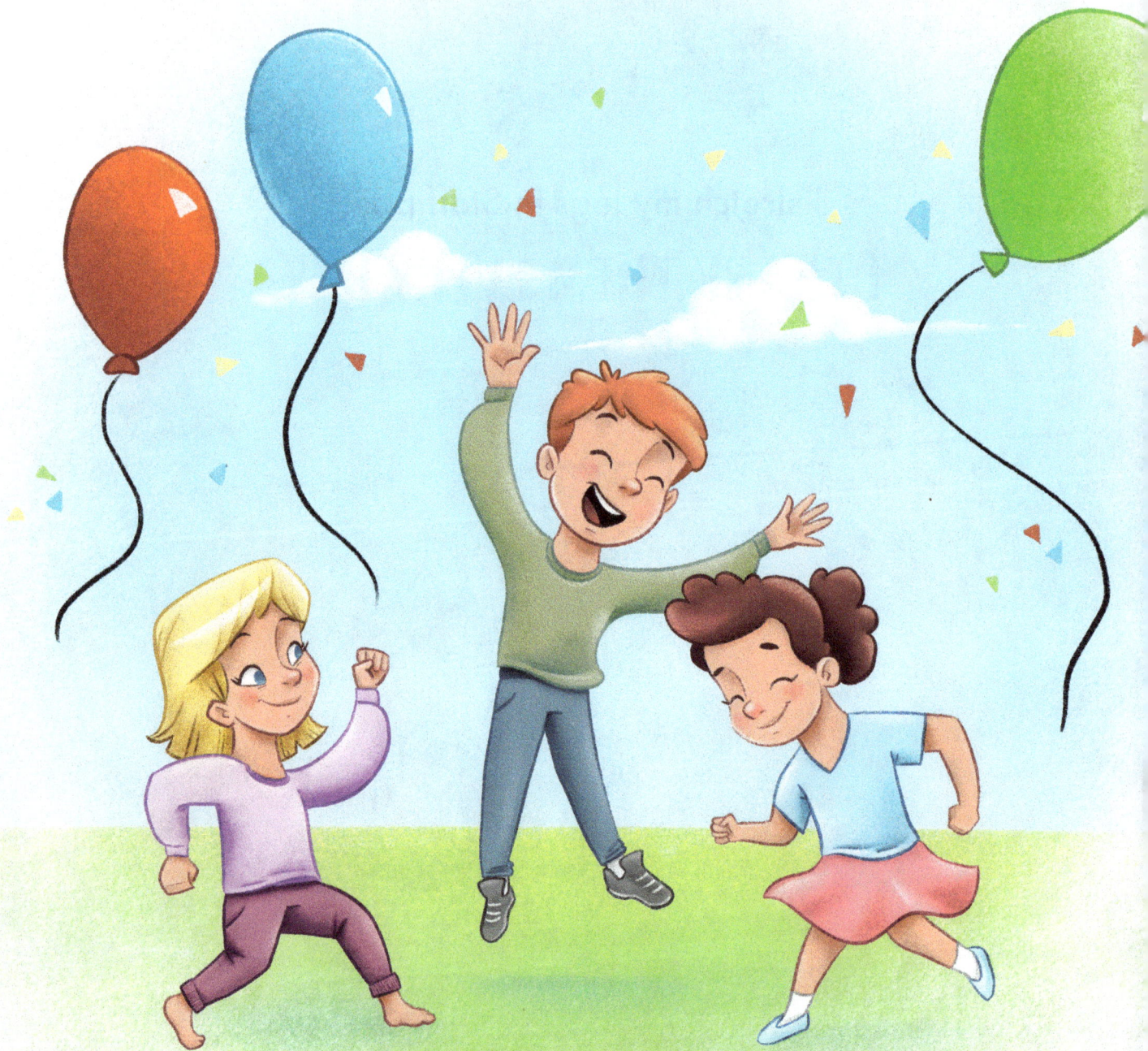

I LOVE MY WIGGLY HIPS ...

when I dance, I feel creative.

I THANK MY HIPS in Frog and Pigeon
for all they have to give.

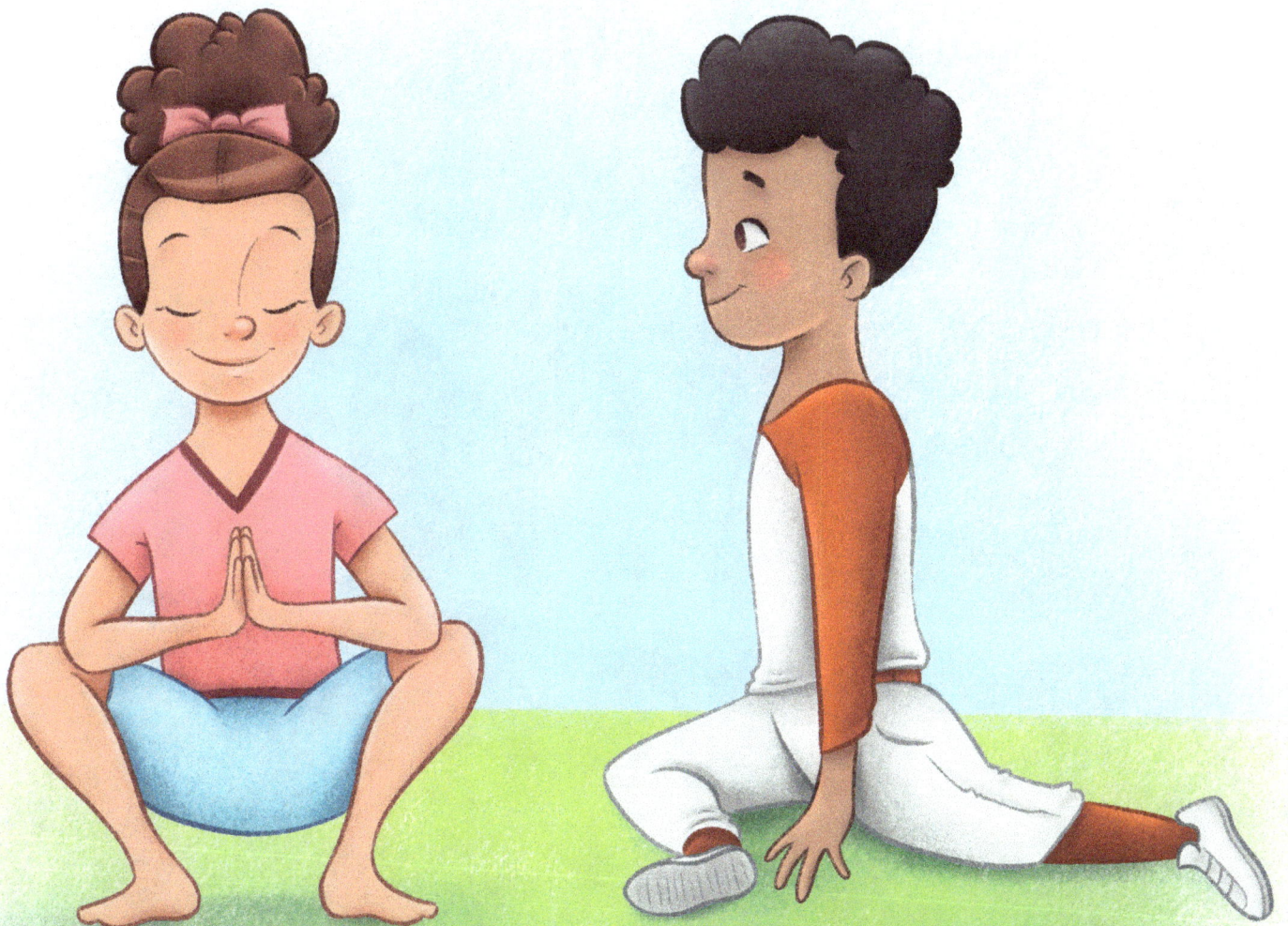

I LOVE MY BACK AND SPINE...

they're how I sit up tall and proud.

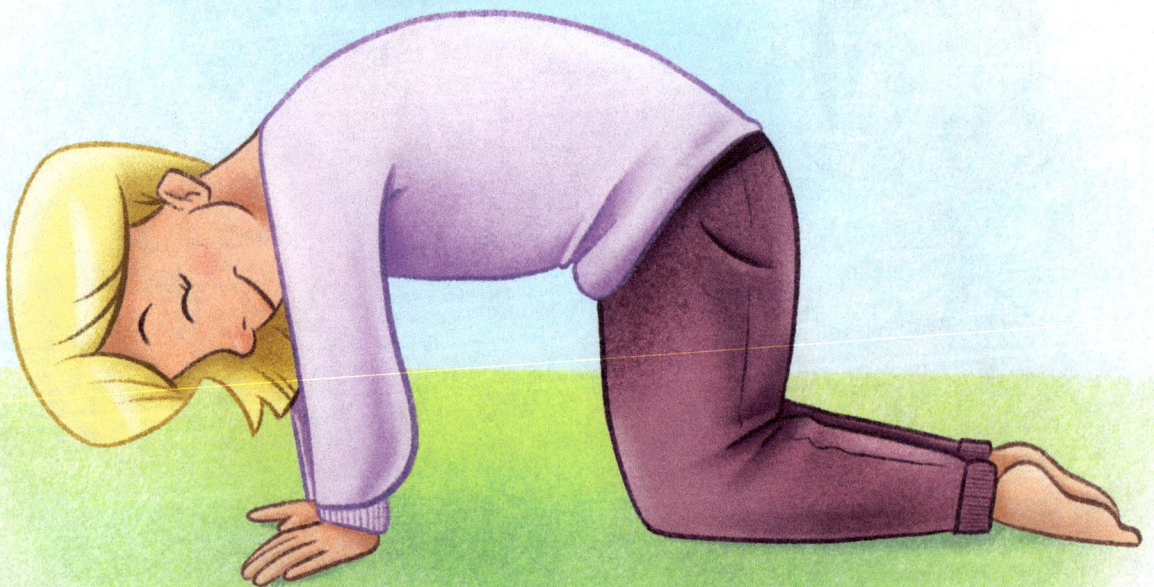

I say **THANK YOU** to my spine
when I'm doing Cats and Cows.

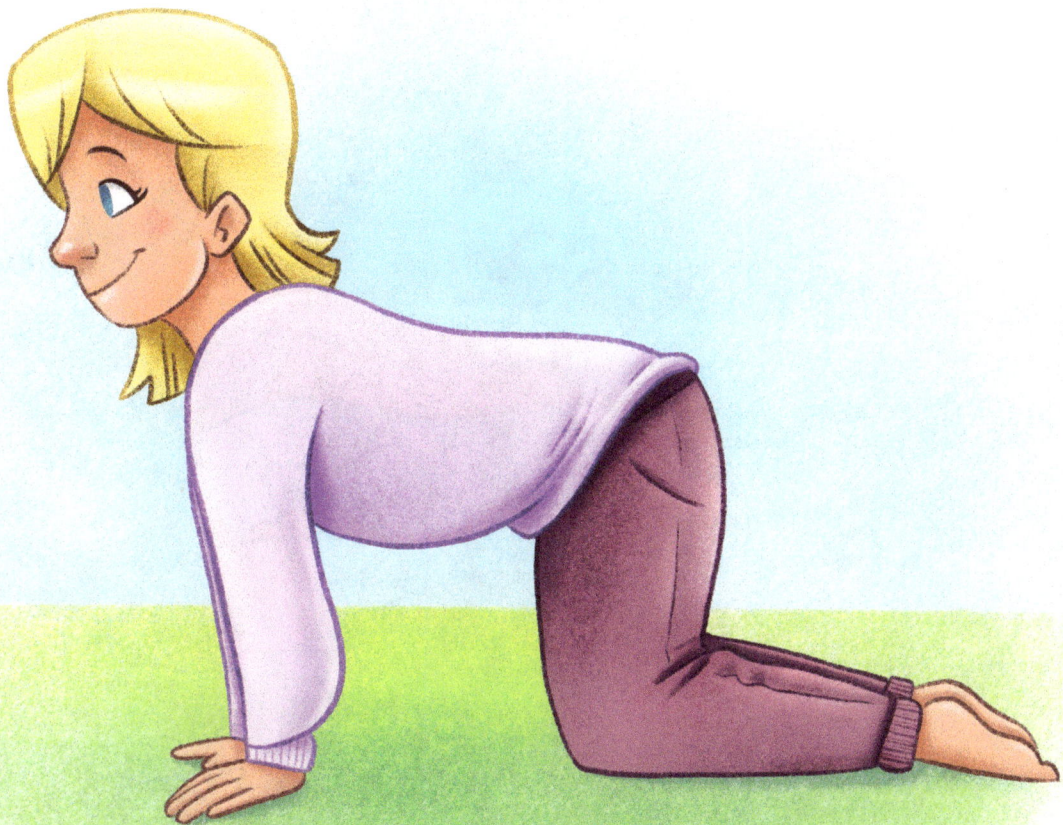

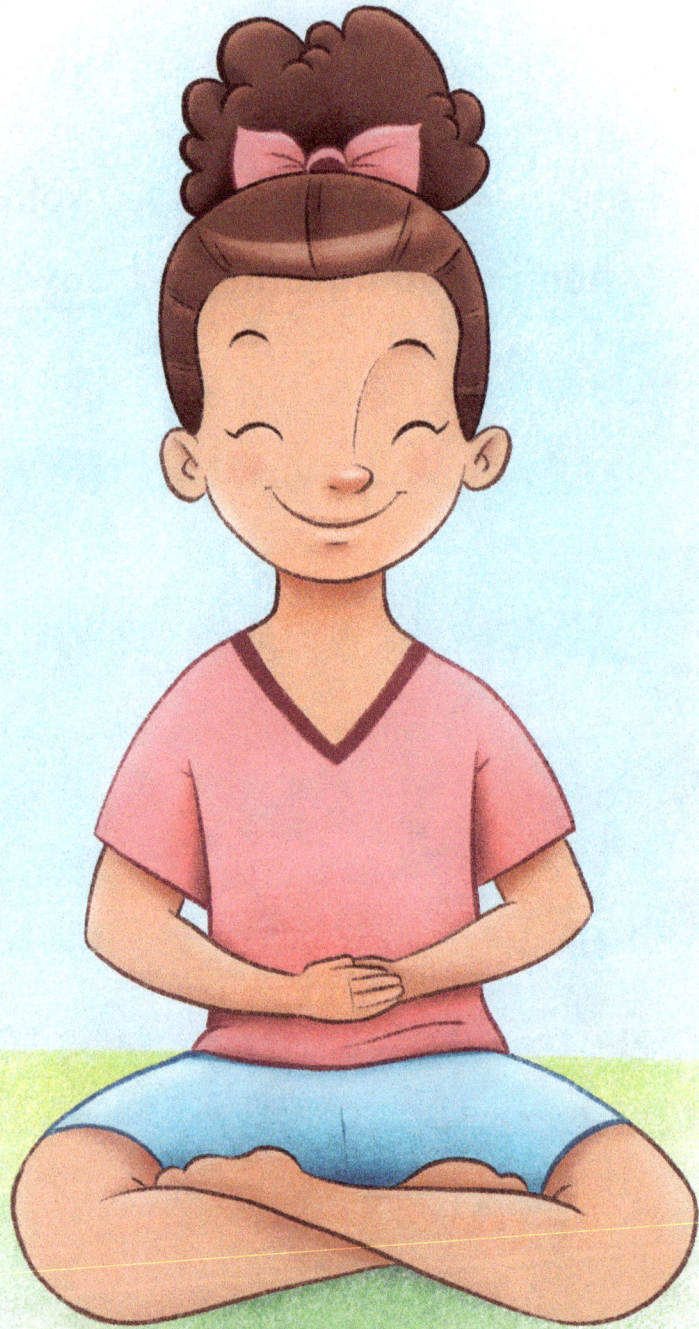

I LOVE MY STRETCHY BELLY ...

it fills up big with air.

I HOLD MY BELLY while I breathe,

to show my belly that I care.

I LOVE MY SHRUGGING SHOULDERS ...

they help me catch and throw.

I say **THANK YOU** to my shoulders

when I breathe in Cobra pose.

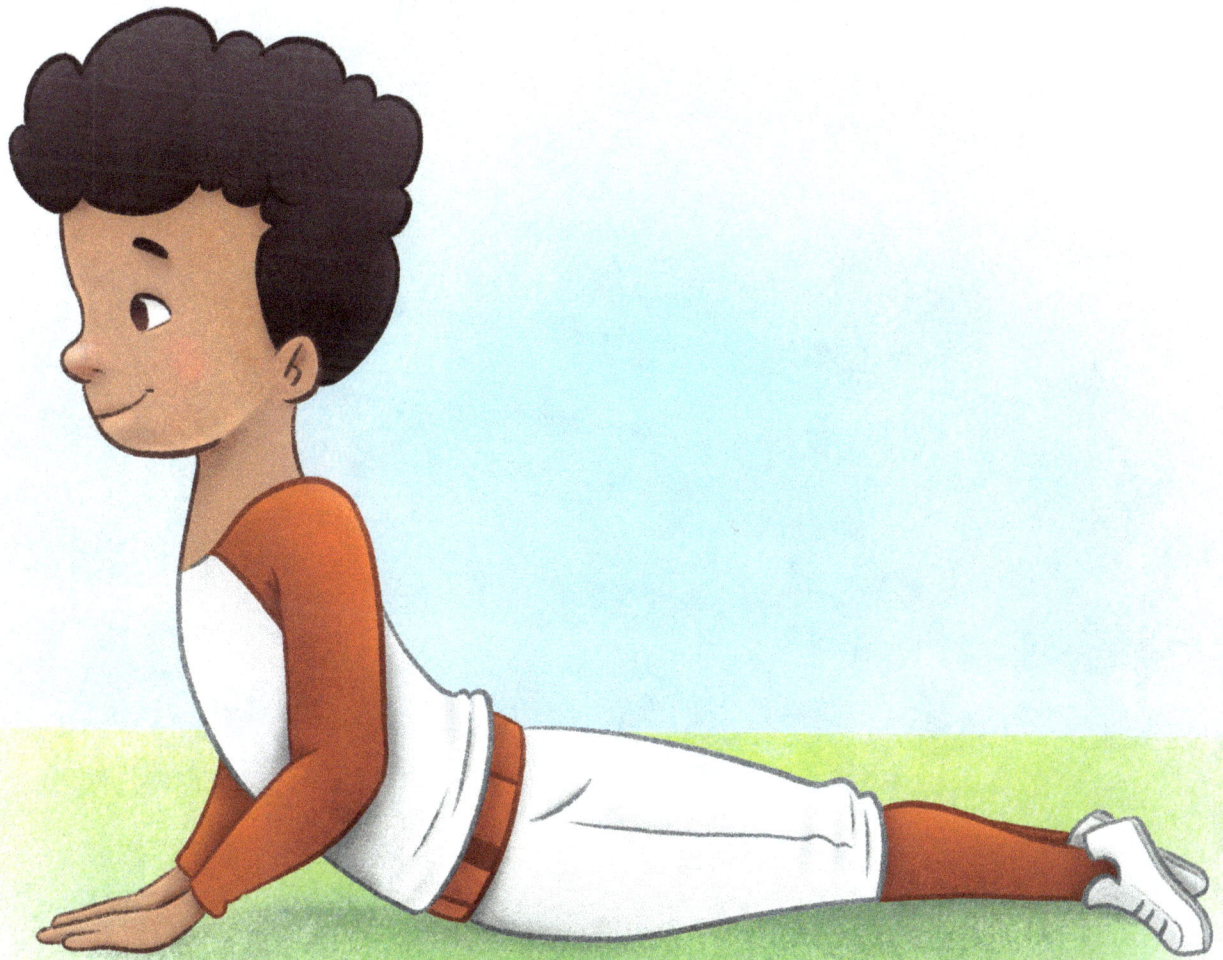

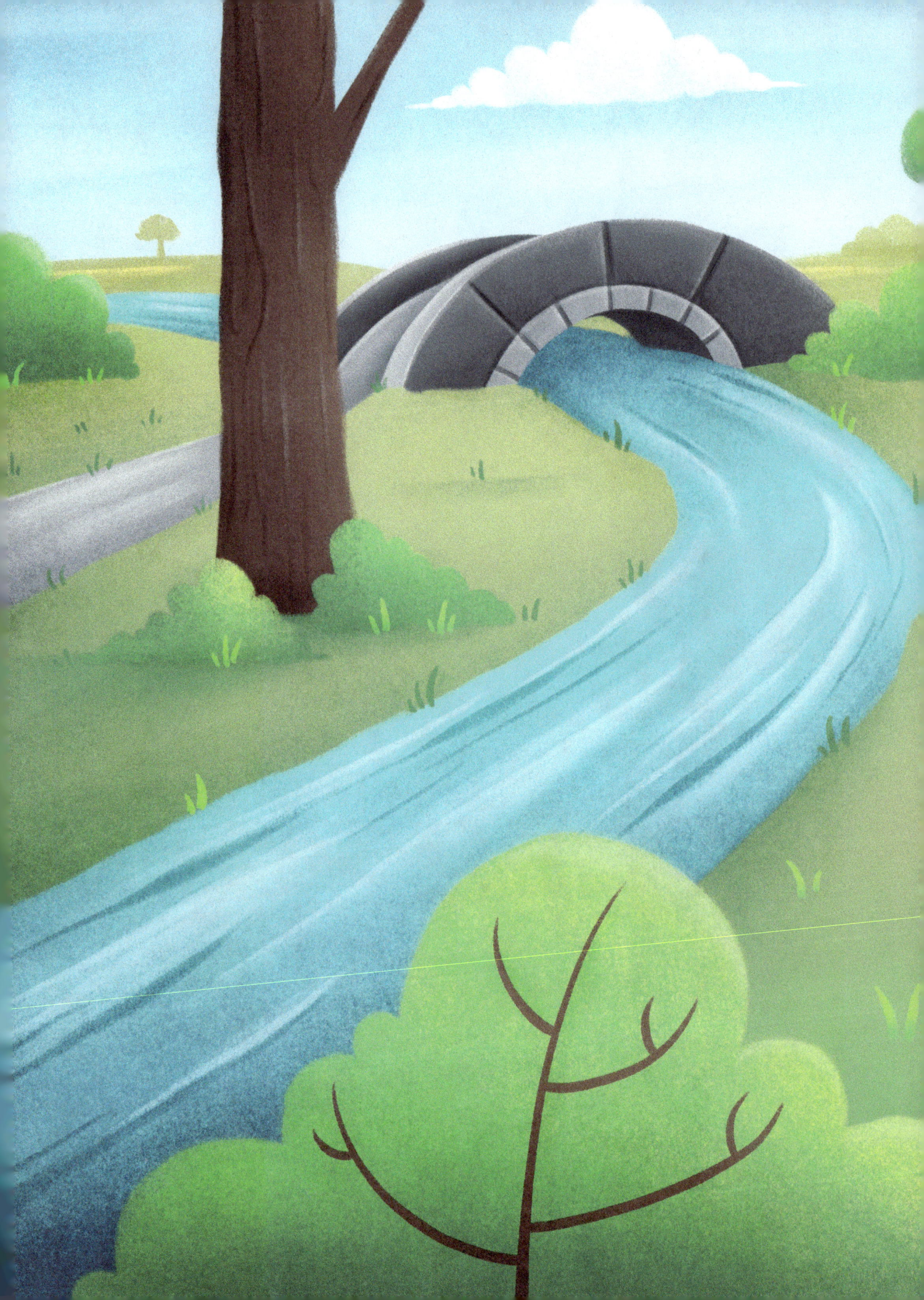

I LOVE MY BIG, KIND HEART . . .
it's where I hold my love.
I THANK MY HEART in Bridge pose,
shoulders down and hips above.

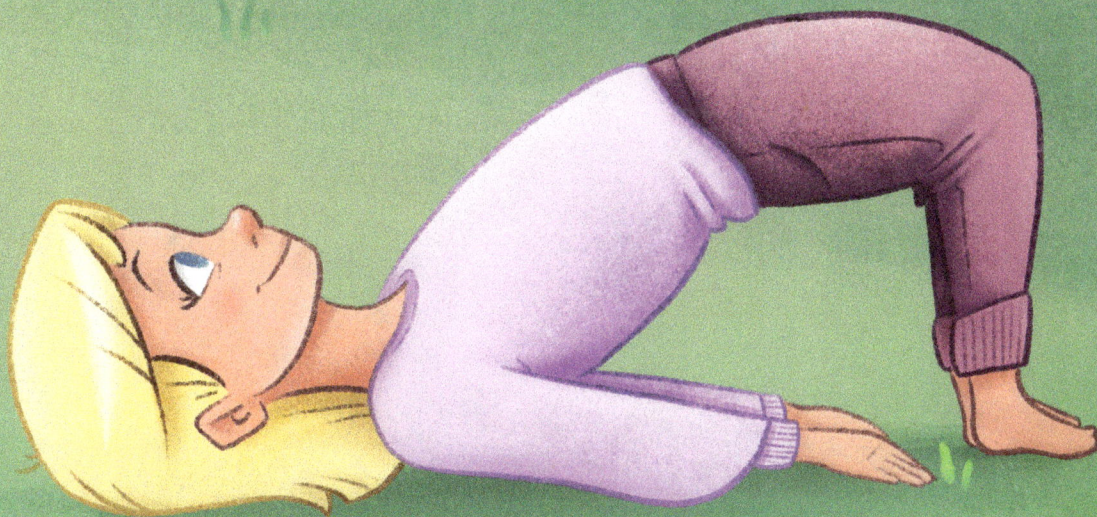

I LOVE MY HANDS AND FINGERS . . .
they do so much for me.
I PUT MY PALMS TOGETHER
and bring them close to me.

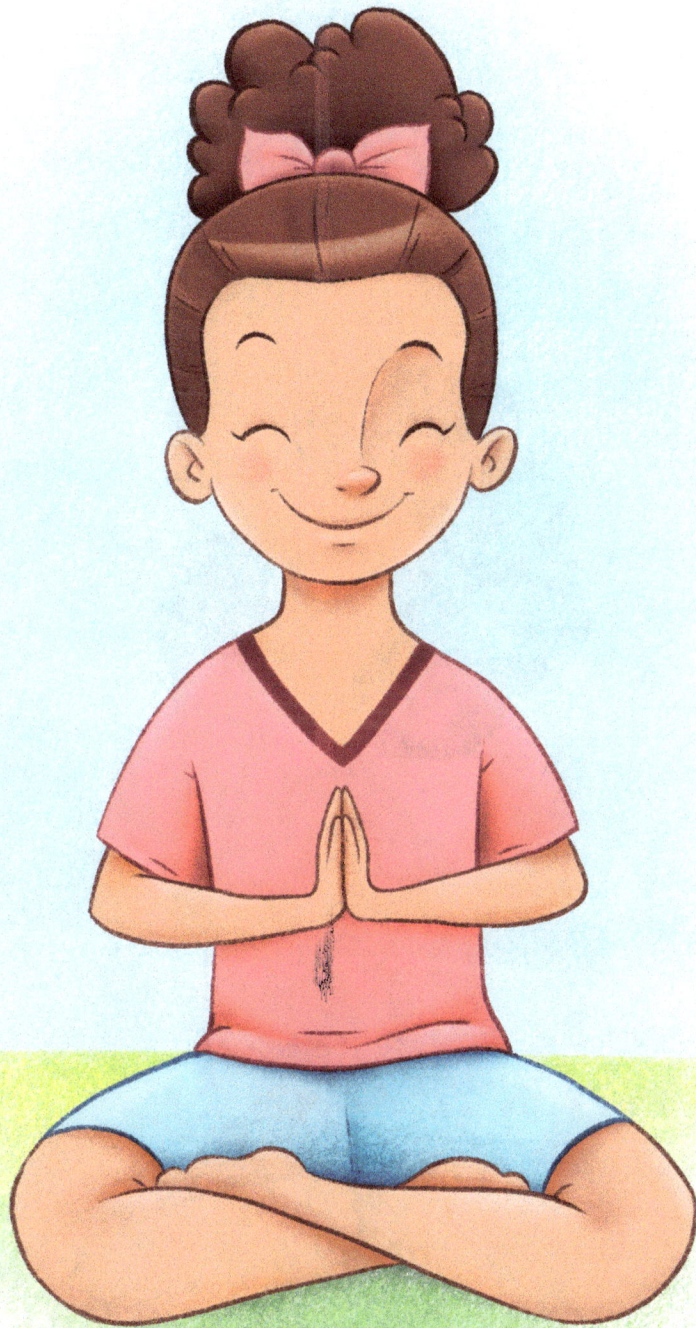

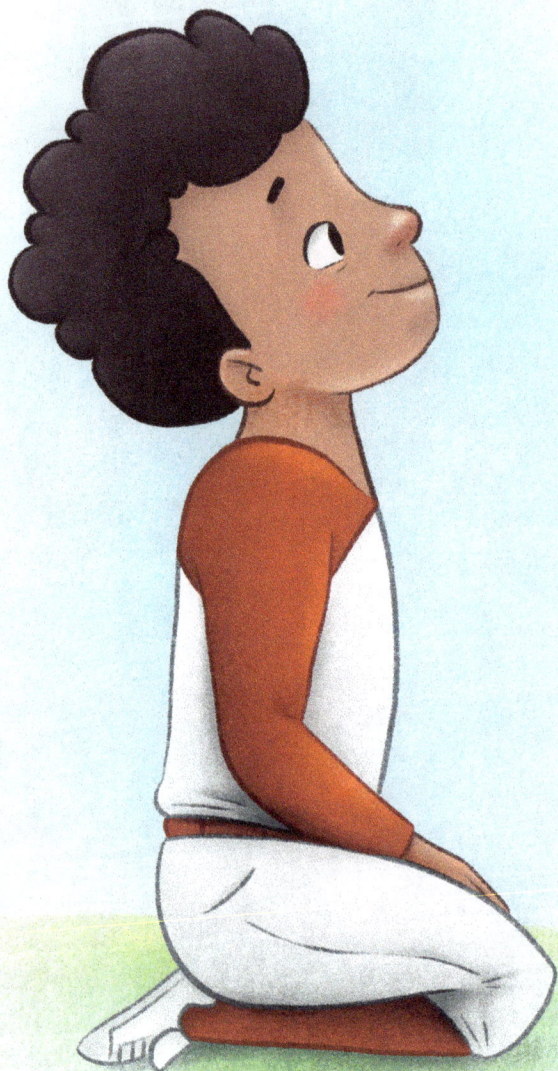

I LOVE MY NECK THAT HOLDS MY HEAD and helps me look around. **I THANK MY NECK** in Thunderbolt— look left, right, up, and down.

I LOVE MY BRILLIANT MIND

for all it does and all it knows.

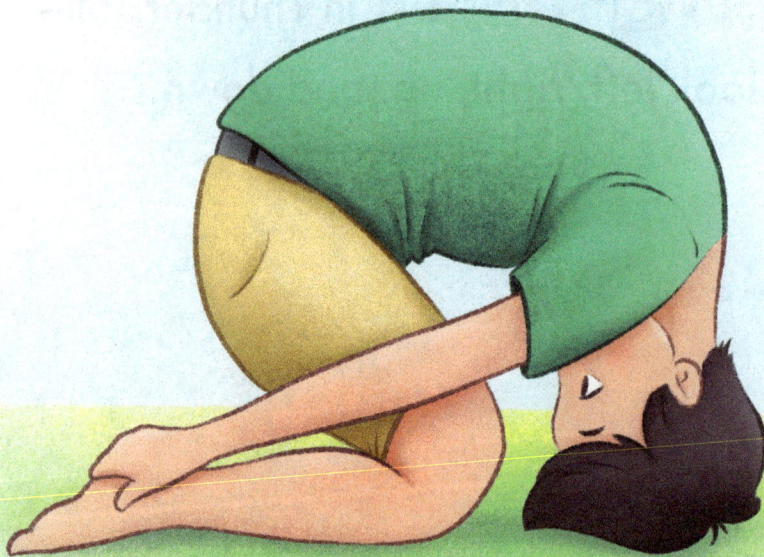

I THANK MY HEAD AND BRAIN

when I practice Rabbit pose.

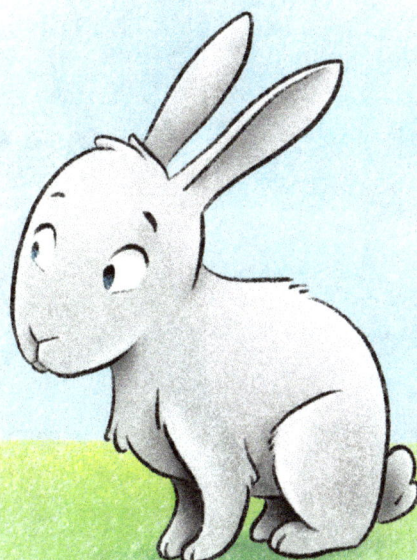

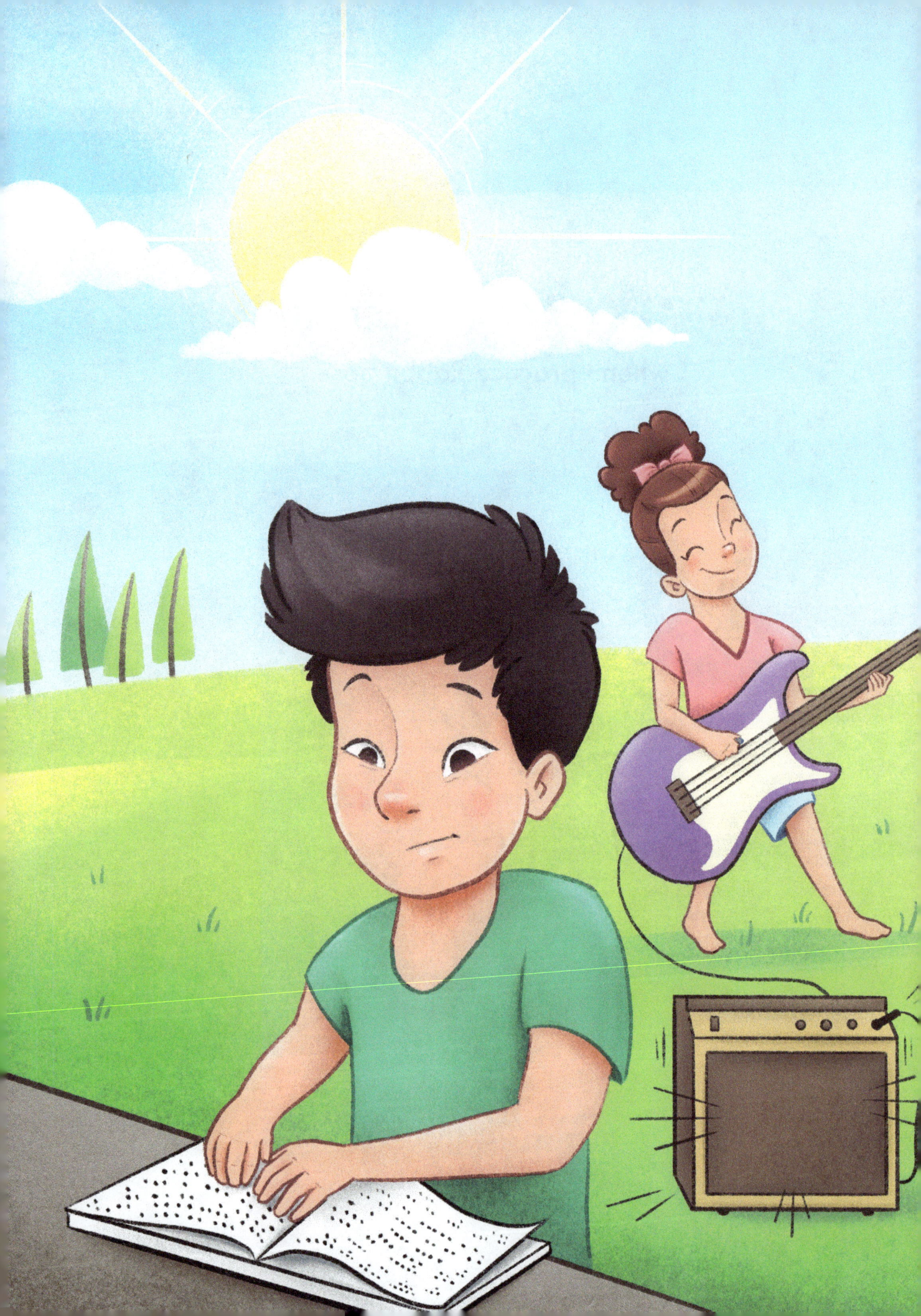

I HAVE SOME SUPERPOWERS . . .

they're sight, smell, touch, taste, and sound.

I THANK MY SENSES for reminding me

I'm in the here and now.

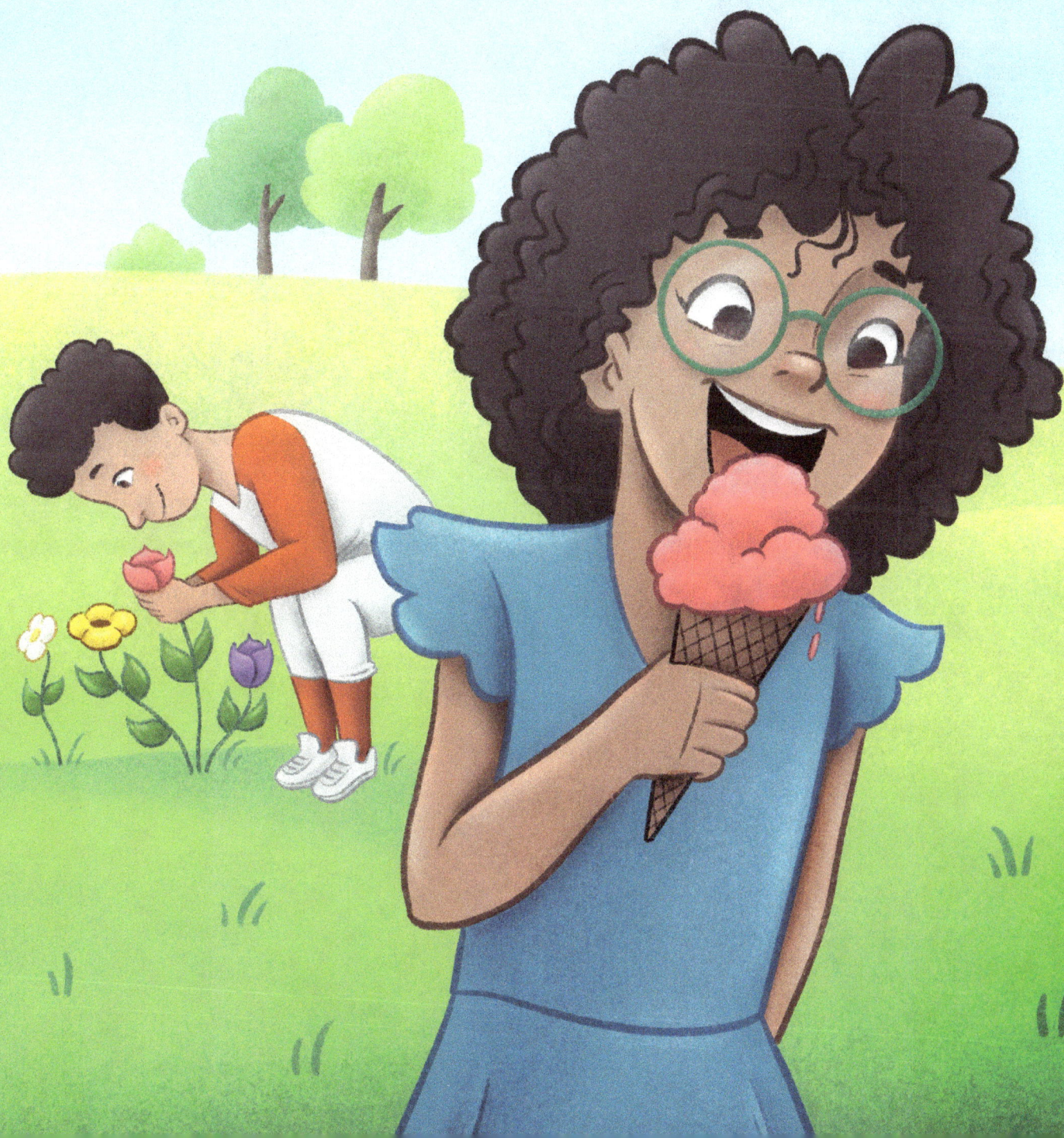

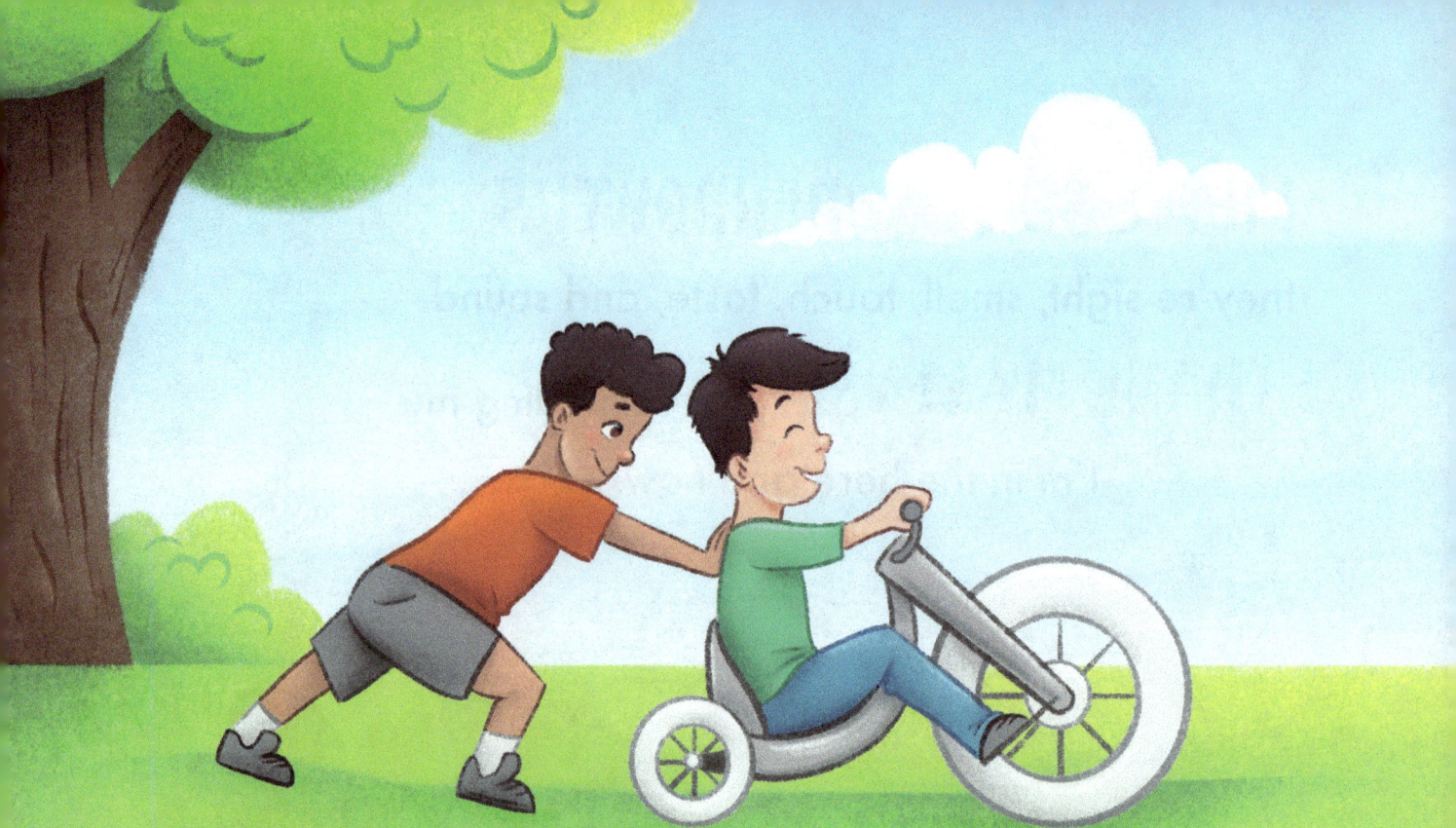

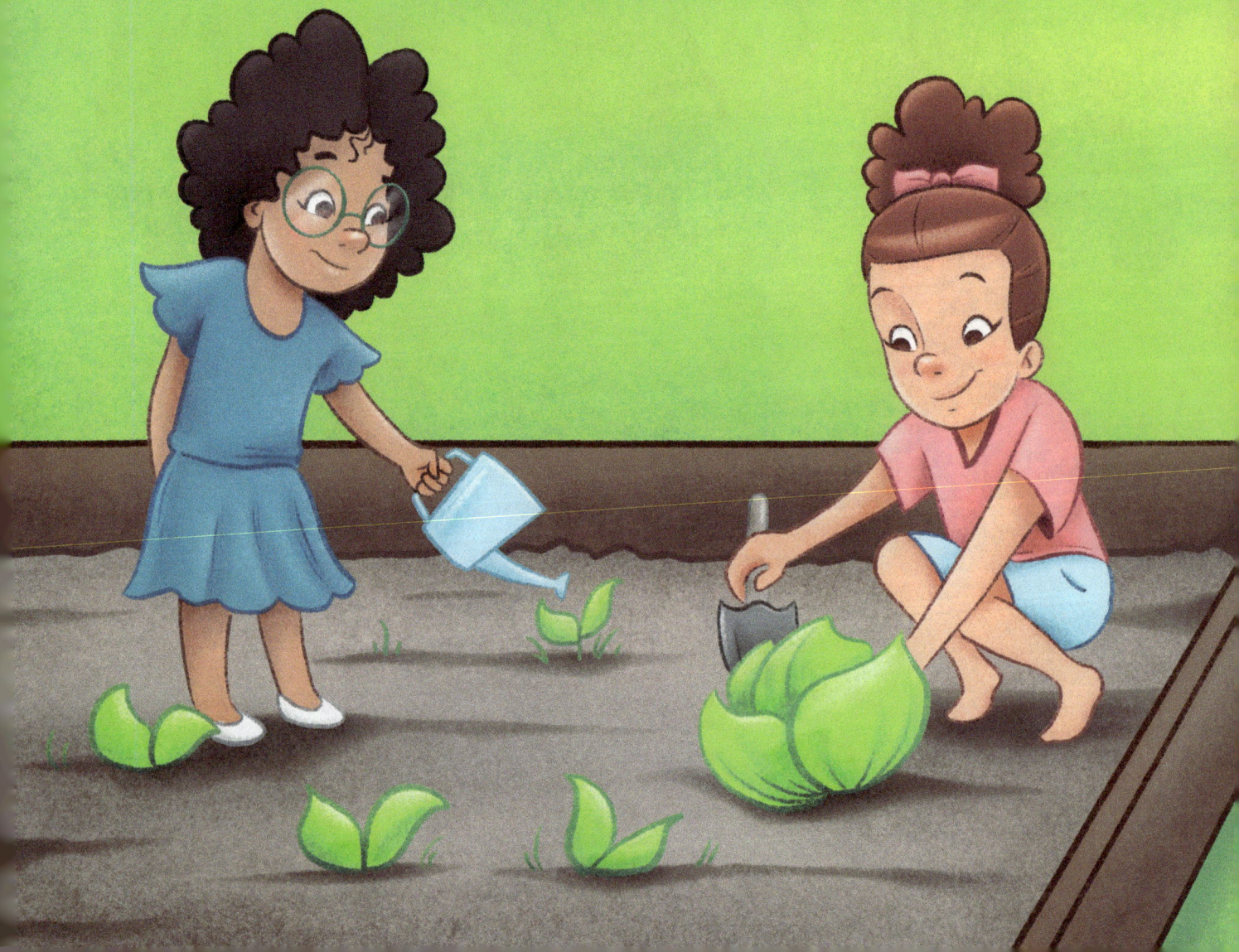

MY BODY IS AMAZING,

but it's not the best part of me.

THE BEST PART isn't even

something you can see.

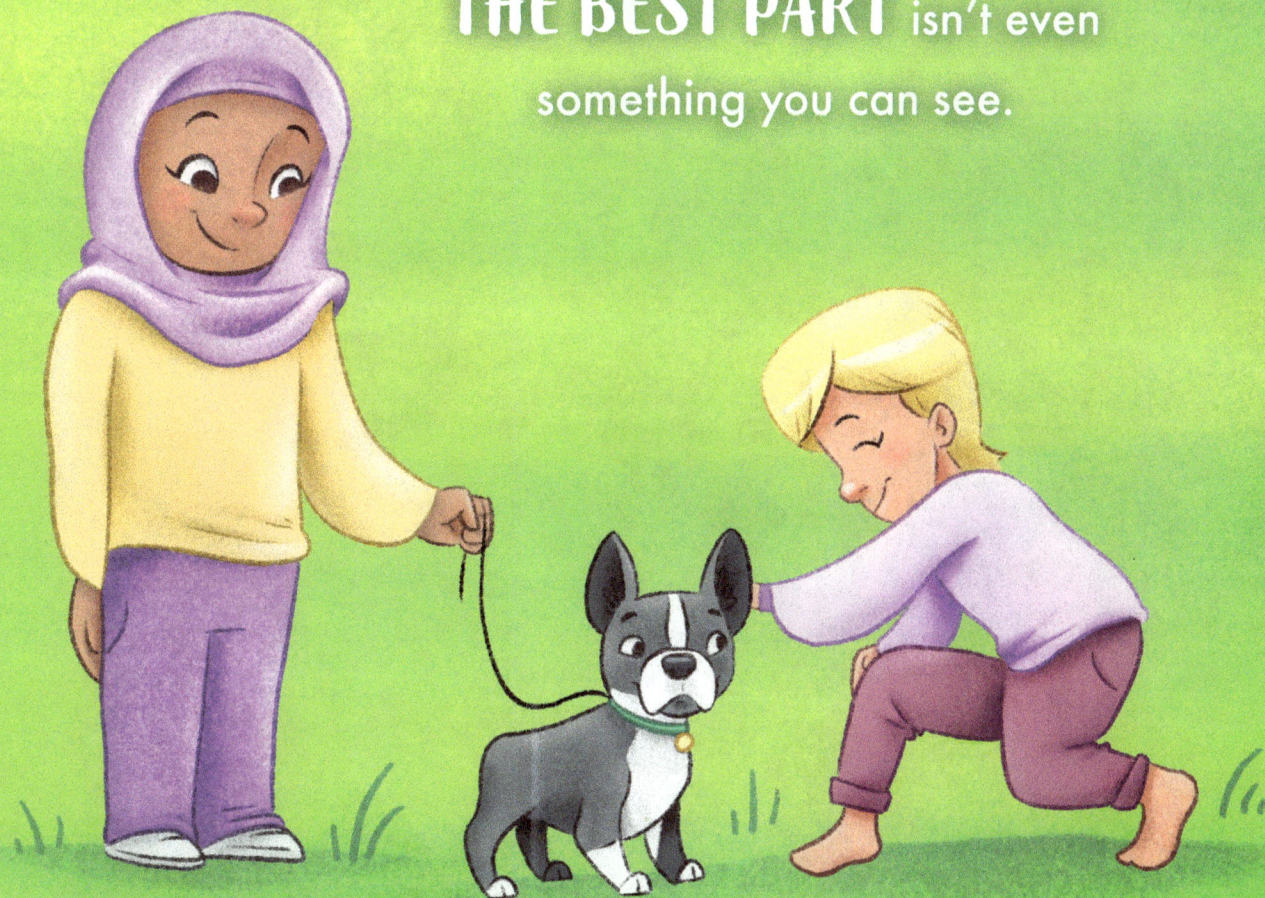

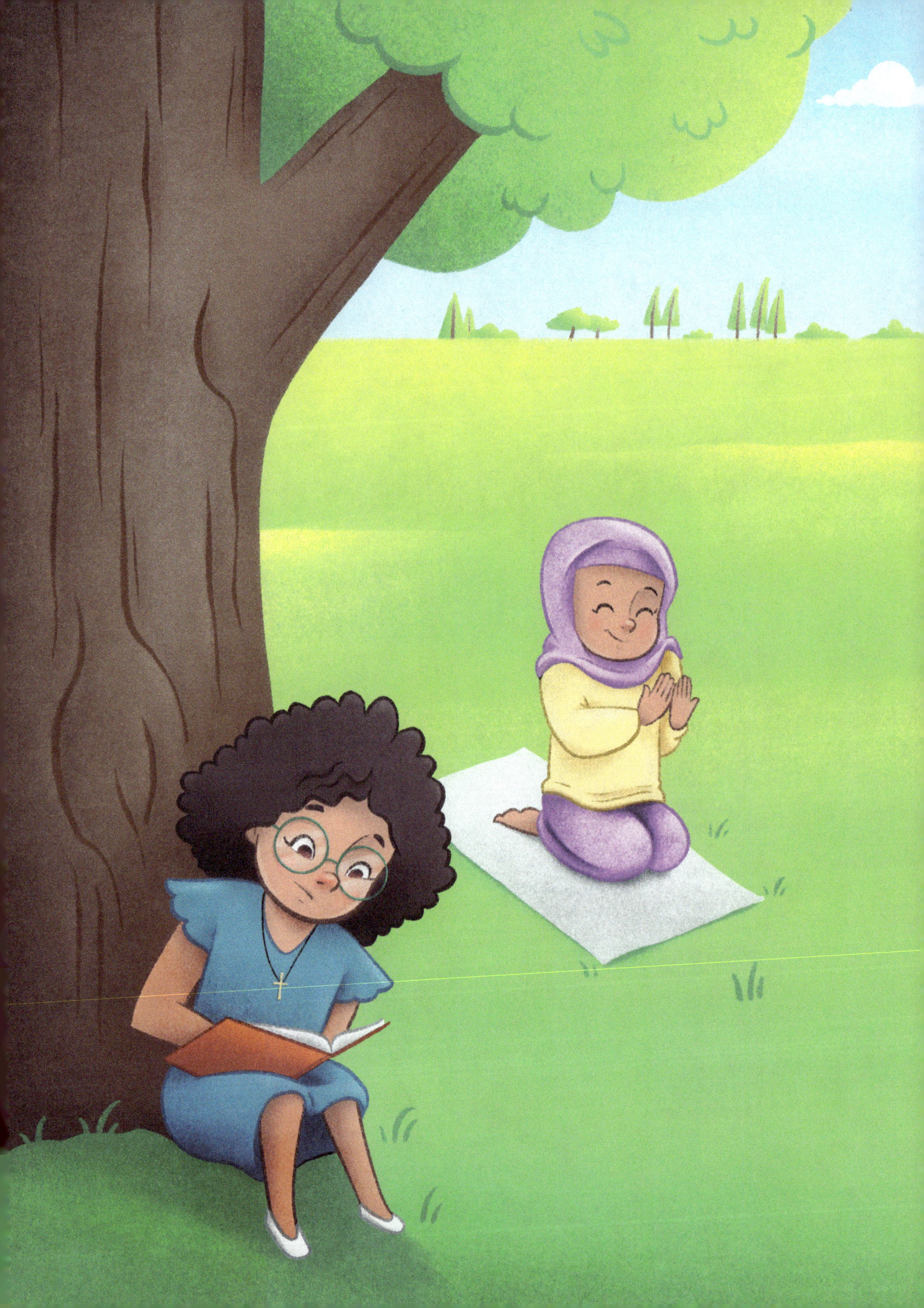

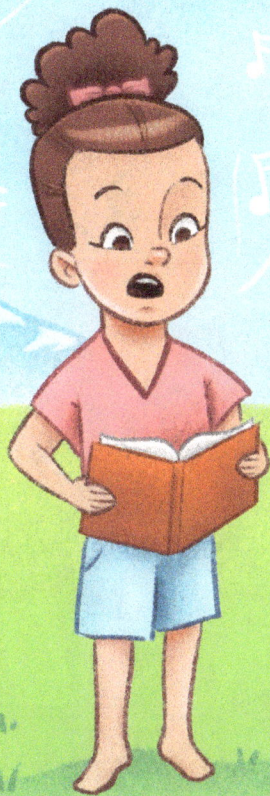

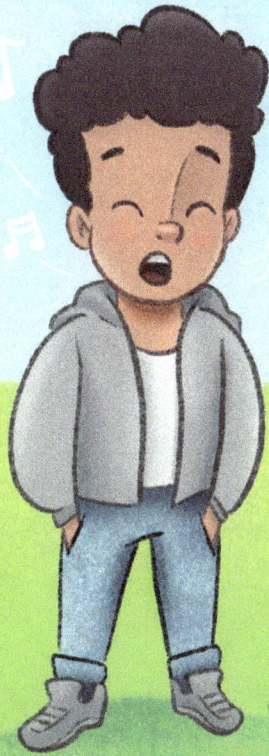

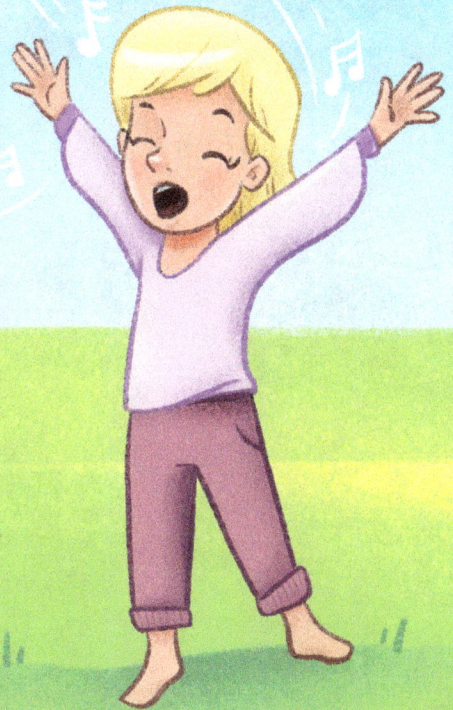

I HAVE A LIGHT within me . . .
it's made of joy and love.
I have gifts and special talents
that are sent from **UP ABOVE.**

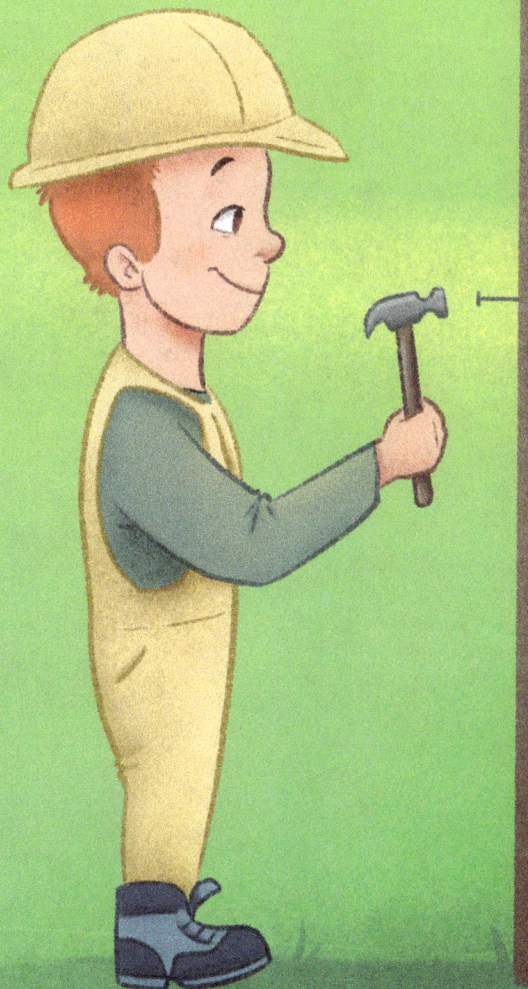

I show **MY LIGHT** to others when I'm being patient, kind, and caring.

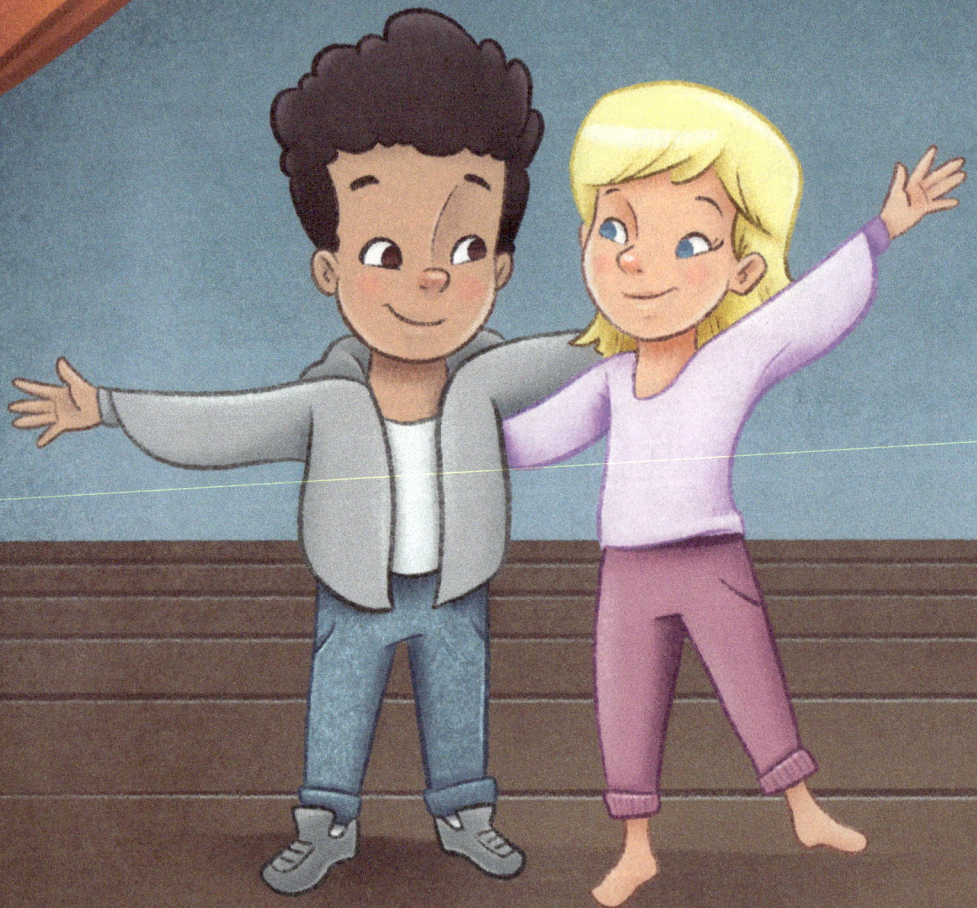

MY LIGHT is meant
to change the world,
my light is meant for sharing.

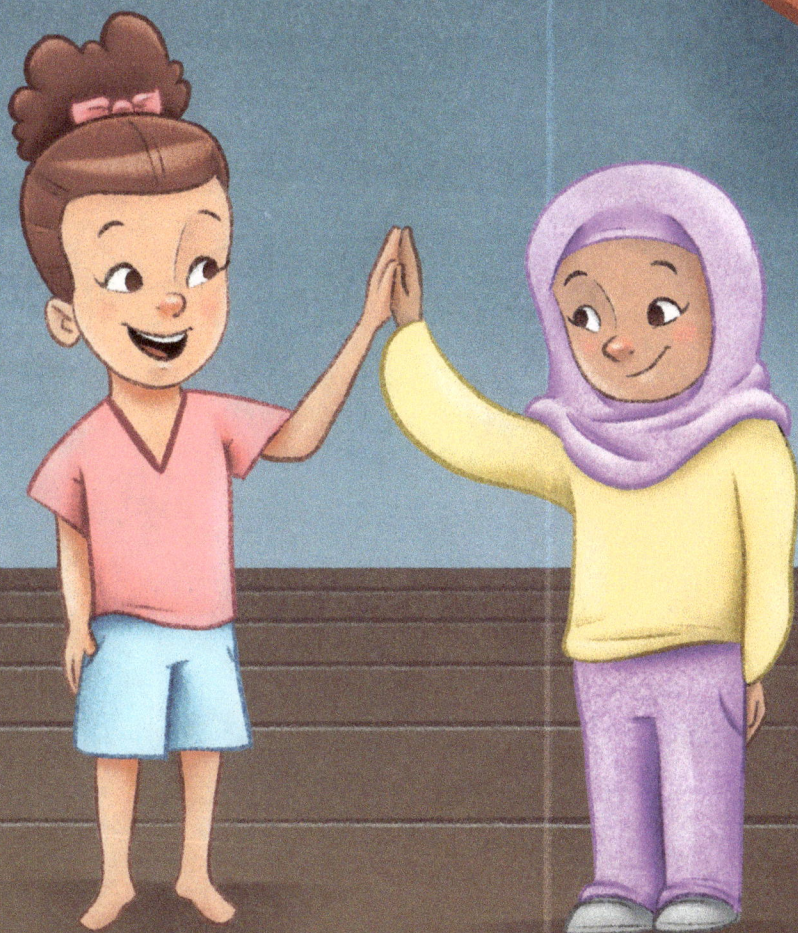

By taking care of me,
my light grows BRIGHTER EVERY DAY.

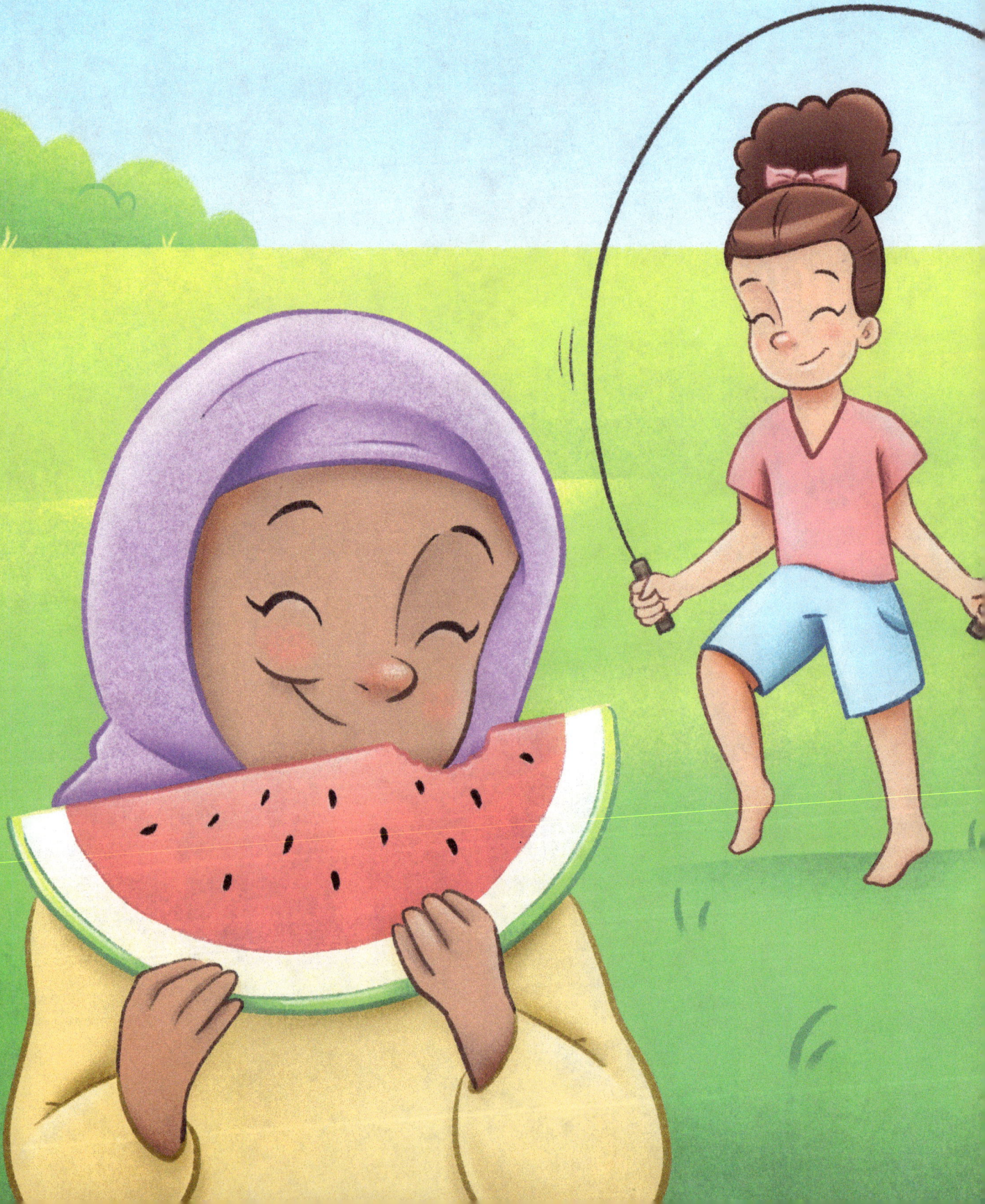

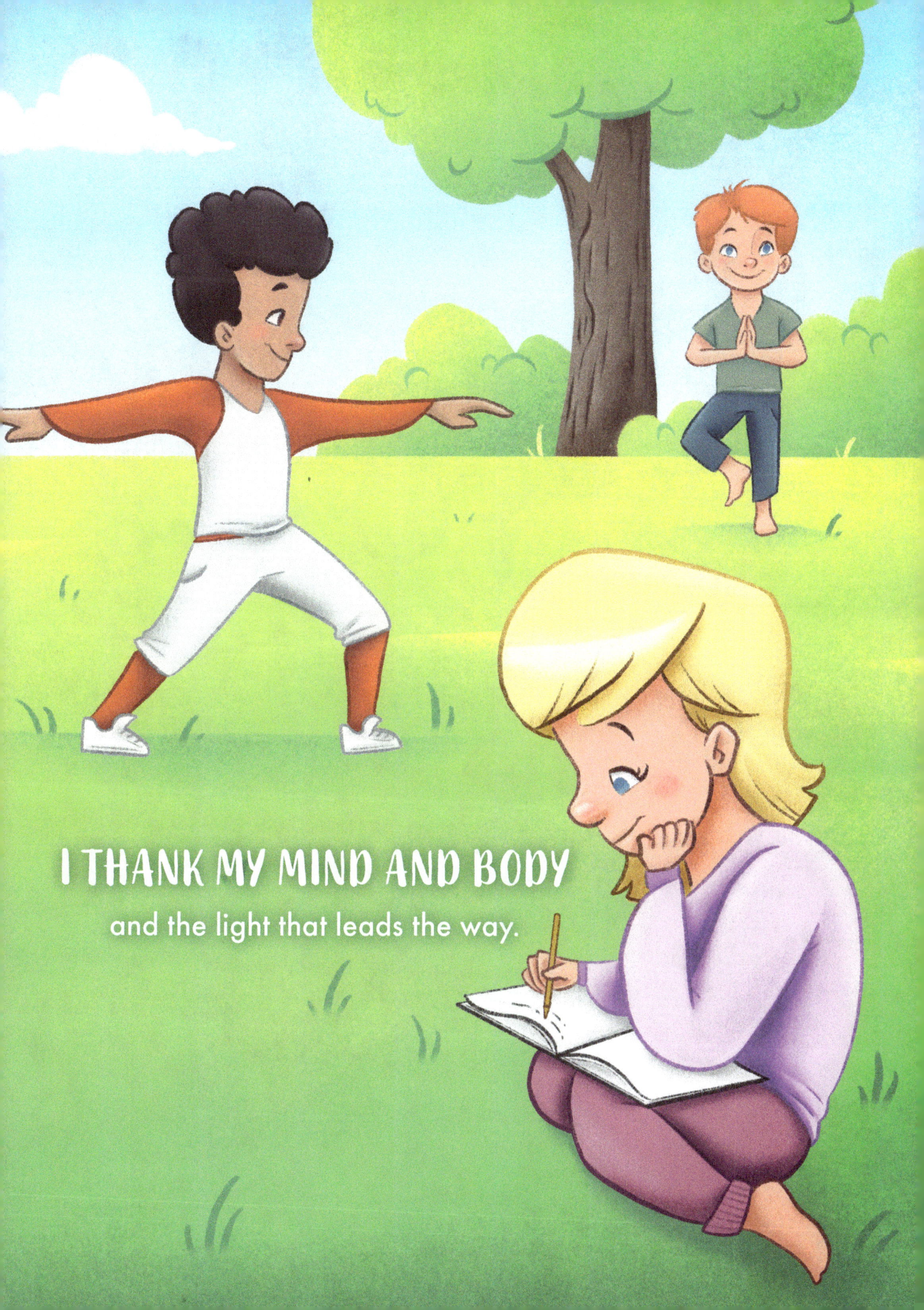

I THANK MY MIND AND BODY

and the light that leads the way.

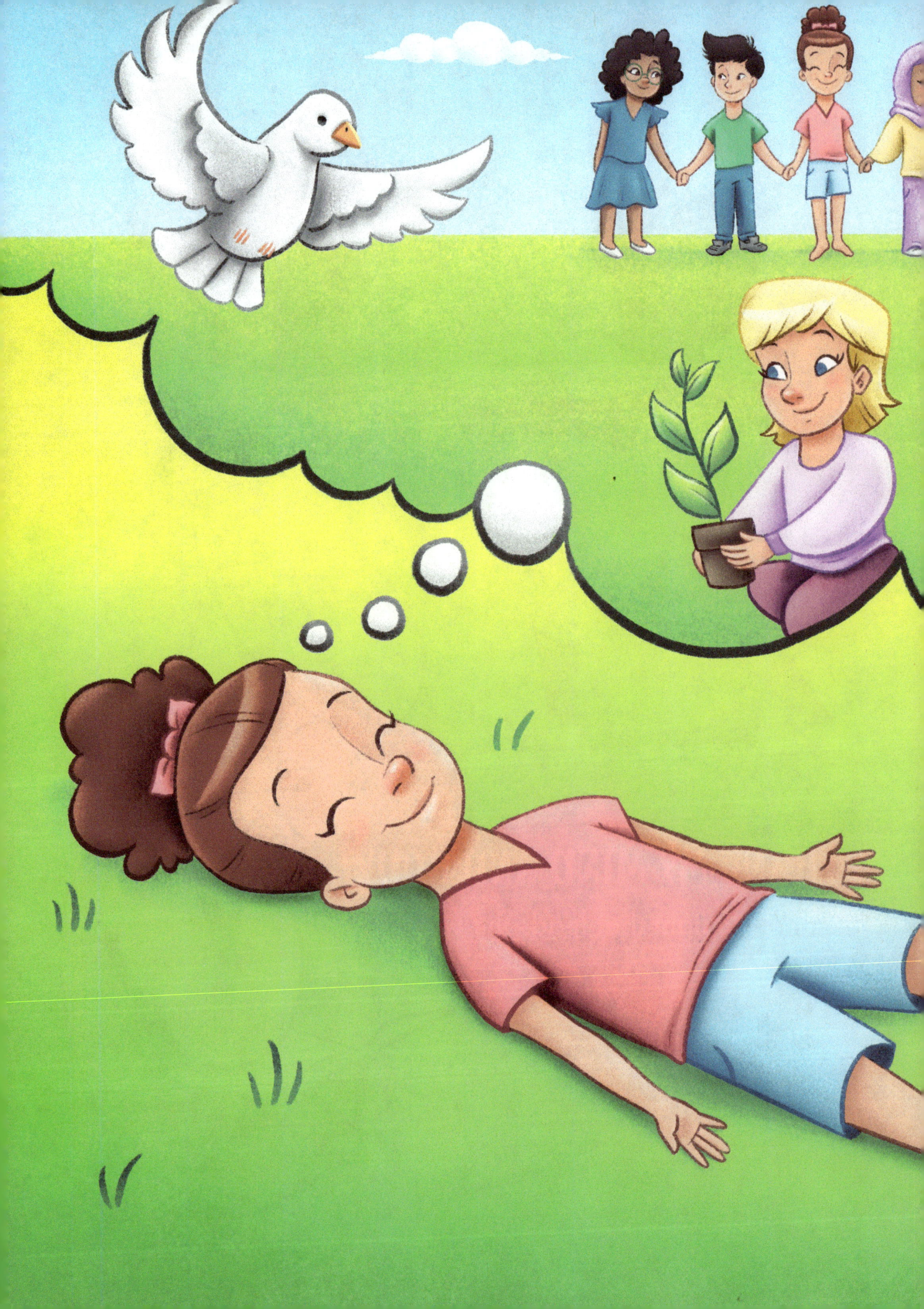

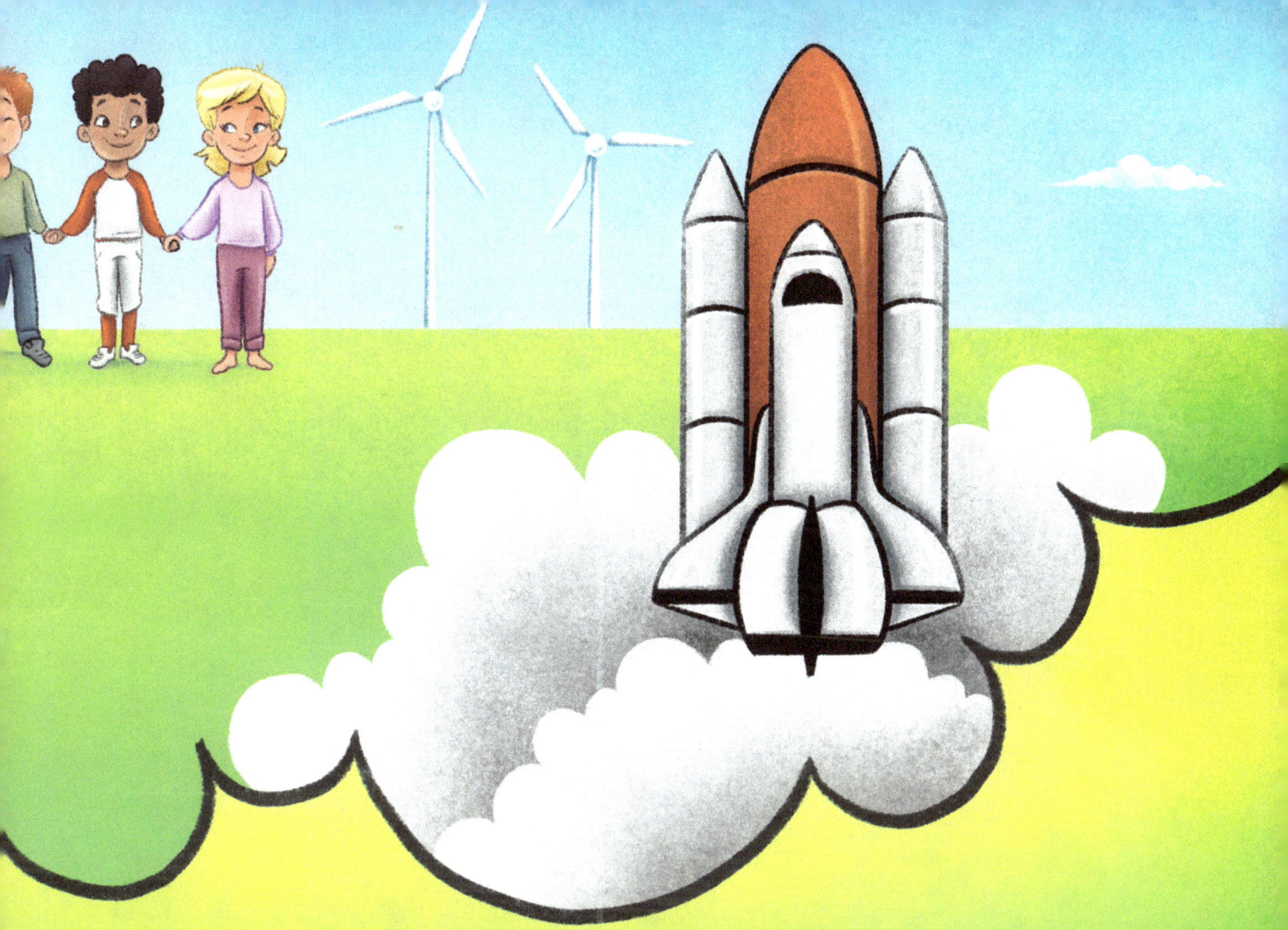

AND SO I SIT IN SILENCE,

breathing in and out through my nose.

BEING ME IS SPECIAL

from my crown down to my toes.

About the Author

Tommie Burch is a certified yoga instructor (RYT-200) with a specialization in prenatal yoga (85-hour) and is also a barre fitness and classical Pilates instructor. Holding a bachelor's degree in early childhood education, Tommie is passionate about fostering self-love, confidence, and a strong mind-body connection in children. As a new mom in 2022, she became even more dedicated to helping the younger generation embrace these transformative practices. Through her platform, Balance by Tommie, she empowers her students to prioritize their well-being and cultivate positive lifestyles through yoga, movement, and breath work. When she's not teaching or hosting yoga retreats, Tommie enjoys reading, working out, and spending time with her family and friends. You can connect with her on Instagram at @balancebytommie or visit her website at www.balancebytommie.com.